VIAGRA (SILD

TREATMENT

Understanding Science of Erectile Dysfunction, Modification of Dopaminergic Pathways And your Problems in Bed.

INCLUDING DOSAGE, SIDE EFFECTS AND ALTERNATIVE METHODS.

Please take your time reading this instruction manual and absorb its contents fully.

Dr. Charles H. Miller

CONTENTS

INTRODUCTION 5

CHAPTER 1 7

THE SCIENCE OF THE HUMAN ERECTION 7

  A Quick Lesson on Sexual Health 7

  Why Do Men Get Erectile Dysfunction? 9

    Circulation 9

    Neurological System 9

    Drugs and Illness 10

    Hormones 10

    Lifestyle 11

  Psychological 13

    Access to Pornography 13

  Debunking Erectile Dysfunction Myths 13

  Erectile Dysfunction Is Caused by Masturbation 14

  Physical Dependence on Viagra Is Inevitable 15

  Erectile Dysfunction Is Something Only Old People Get 15

  Infertility and erectile dysfunction are synonymous. 16

  Erectile Dysfunction Is an AZZ or Nothing Phenomenon 16

CHAPTER 2 18

THE HISTORY OF TREATING ERECTILE DYSFUNCTION 18

  Wacky "Cures" for Not Getting It Up 18

CHAPTER 3 21

WHAT 15 VIAGRA AND HOW DOES IT WORK? 21

  Obtaining a Prescription 21

  Contraindications 22

The Viagra Alternative 23

What Viagra Is Not... 24

Your marriage may not be saved by this. 25

CHAPTER 4 27

THINGS YOU SHOULD KNOW BEFORE TAKING VIAGRA 27

Common Side Effects of Viagra 27

Negative Repercussions That Can Occur Very Infrequently 28

Vision Loss 28

Loss of Hearing 28

"If Your Erections Lasts for More Than Four Hours, Seek Medical
Attention Immediately" 29

Contraindications and Interactions between Drugs 29

Other Interactions 30

Alcohol 30

Grapefruit 31

CHAPTER 5 32

OTHER FACTORS THAT CAN IMPROVE ERECTILE DYSFUNCTION......... 32

Exercise 32

Diet 32

Therapy 33

To Liven Up Your Sexual Experience 33

Options to Viagra 34

CONCLUSION 36

INTRODUCTION

The 65-year-old Jeremy is at his urologist's office, reading a cookery magazine nervously. His head is a black hole filled with anxiety, shame, and rage. His wife had finally suggested he consult a doctor, and he couldn't believe it. For a while now, Jeremy has had trouble getting an erection.

Throughout their thirty-year marriage, he took great joy in making her happy. Initially, it was quite challenging to maintain. That was the problem, but now he has lost the ability to have an erection altogether. To confide in another person about a problem he should be able to handle on his own made him feel like a failure. His sense of manhood had been shattered, and he was terrified that his wife would blame herself or that the doctor would tell him there was nothing they could do. But he was at a loss and feared going into the clinic for his scheduled visit. Outside of his field of vision, he noticed a younger man, perhaps in his mid-20s, and pondered why he was seeing an urologist.

While waiting to see his new urologist, Matt stared into space, scrolled mindlessly, and checked social media on his phone. Humbled beyond words, he could not believe he had to watch someone so young. Like Matt, you probably spent the day in the office because you're having problems in your sex life. His inability to develop and keep an erection led to several less-than-desirable one-night hookups. Matt couldn't wrap his brain around it; he'd always assumed these kinds of problems only arose in the elderly, not healthy men in their twenties. Matt's inability to perform in bed was a self-fulfilling prophecy: every time he tried to have sex, he thought about the occasions when he had failed. While some of the ladies were able to get past his mistake and offer words of comfort, others could not hide their dismay. Friends who lied about him would brag about their successful sex life, and he would have to listen in envy. One day, he went on a date with a nurse who recommended he consult an urologist. Matt had not even graduated from his parents' health insurance plan when he found himself waiting in an office to discuss eating disorder treatment.

Despite coming from opposite generations, these two men have identical problems. Predicting if someone has ED just by looking at them is not possible. Many different kinds of people can be affected by this for many different reasons. There are a variety of approaches that can be used to treat ED in males, and these vary depending on the underlying causes.

It takes courage to admit you have Erectile Dysfunction (ED) and look for treatment options. You should feel proud that you are making progress toward normalcy if this is a challenge for you. Increasing percentages of males are experiencing this problem. The actual number of men who struggle with erectile dysfunction is likely higher than the thirty million who have admitted to needing help. As a matter of fact, only approximately 30% of men who experience ED will seek professional care, especially if it is an inconsistent problem. There are many possible treatments to this problem, however the pill most commonly mentioned is Sildenafil (which is what the brand name Viagra is) or Viagra (trade name) (generic name). When asked directly about their pharmaceutical use, most men are unlikely to speak up, even when the topic is otherwise safe. Consequently, males may not be informed of the truth about the pill. If you've been prescribed Viagra, you probably have a lot of questions, from the proper dosage and list of possible side effects to drug interactions and further treatments for erectile dysfunction (ED). Learning about Viagra, erectile dysfunction, and your own biology is essential for success in treating ED.

CHAPTER 1

THE SCIENCE OF THE HUMAN ERECTION

A QUICK LESSON ON SEXUAL HEALTH

The male sexual organs consist of several different parts.

- The penis consists of a shaft and a head; it is the primary sexual organ.

- Sperm is stored in the testicles. They can fold in or fall depending on the surrounding conditions.

- Located midway up the penis, the corpus cavernosa consists of two chambers. When blood fills these cavities, an erection results.

- Finally, there is the urethra that carries semen and urine out of the body.

There are two main types of erections: reflex and psychogenic. Penal tumescence in response to random or nonspecific touch constitutes a reflex. Teenagers who have become tense in the middle of math class will understand this concept all too well. Similar to the way your hand instinctively moves away from flames, this process relies solely on the spinal nerves rather than your brain. An ordinary reflex loop. It's also the reason why some guys get nighttime erections.

A psychogenic erection is one that is brought on by mental processes rather than physical ones, such as through sensory stimulation or fantasizing. The brain can be triggered to release a flood of hormones that travel down the spine to inhibit the nerves that prevent erections and stimulate the nerves that induce it by means of sight, smell, sound, and sexually stimulating contact.

The human erection is controlled by the parasympathetic nervous system, the branch of the nervous system that is supposed to let you relax, even though arousal is a stimulating feeling. Think about it: if our ancestors were being followed by a wolf, being horny wouldn't have helped. When the parasympathetic signal reaches the penis, it has the same effect regardless of its origin. The pelvis is the site of a cascade of metabolic events that, once initiated, translate the signal into an actual effect. Vasodilation, or the widening of blood vessels, occurs when nitric oxide (NO) is produced inside the body's cells. This allows more blood to flow into the corpus cavernosa. Keep in mind that this does not lead to skeletal muscle relaxation (the muscles you control to move). Muscle relaxation and vasodilation are aided by the release of cyclic guanosine monophosphate, which opens and closes potassium and ion channels in the penis's muscles. All of these factors contribute to a prolonged erection by allowing the corpora cavernosa to fill with blood and trap it.

In a perfect world, a man would ejaculate to release the tension. The vas deferanse in the testicle transports sperm from the testicles to the urethra during the peak of sexual activity. The man builds up pressure and ejaculates quickly, like a shot. Dopamine, oxytocin, and other endorphins flood the brain, making you feel extremely happy.

Arousal, erection, orgasm, and ejaculation are often confused with one another or thought to occur simultaneously because of this. To get an erection, arousal is not required. You don't need have to ejaculate to get some relief from an erection. As a matter of fact, orgasms can occur without ejaculating at all (this would be a dry orgasm). Most men have a full-body sensation called an orgasm, which includes their brain, genitalia, and strong muscle contractions. This facilitates human bonding, which has evolutionary benefits. Due to the lengthier gestation period of female animals and the helplessness of human infants for extended periods of time, this link is crucial. When males cared about their families, they were better able to safeguard their pregnant partners and their offspring. This confusion contributes to the over-hyped status of ED treatments, which can lead to disillusionment with these drugs in the future.

WHY DO MEN GET ERECTILE DYSFUNCTION?

The erection itself is a multisystem function, hence the underlying cause of ED may be complex. Many different factors can contribute to ED. A problem with blood flow is usually to blame. Erectile dysfunction (ED) has several potential causes, including one's way of life, other diseases, medications or treatments (particularly for prostate cancer), any disturbance to the neurological system, or even psychological disorders.

CIRCULATION

Blood flow problems are the leading cause of erectile dysfunction. Keep in mind that a lot of blood needs to flow into the penis for an erection to occur. Reduced systemic blood flow can be caused by a number of factors, including a weak heart or clogged arteries. Complications such as heart disease, high blood pressure (although having a high blood pressure reading does not necessarily mean that it is high in the proper locations), and excessive cholesterol should be considered while treating erectile dysfunction. To avoid ED, it is recommended to maintain a healthy heart through regular exercise. True, ED is a potent indicator of future cardiovascular problems. Loss of erection stability is an early indicator of deteriorating heart condition. Visit both a cardiologist and a urologist for a thorough examination of the cardiovascular system.

NEUROLOGICAL SYSTEM

As the erection is triggered by a nerve signal traveling to the penis, damage to those nerves or disruptions in the signal can result in erectile dysfunction (ED). There is no way for the body to know it should release NO to dilate the arteries in the absence of the signal. As a result of the injury to the spinal cord, patients typically experience ED. Nonetheless,

ED can be brought on by neuropathy from diabetes or other neurological disorders including Parkinson's, ALS, or MS (MS).

DRUGS AND ILLNESS

The unfortunate reality is that some of the medicines we take may have unintended consequences in the bedroom. One side effect of painkillers is a slow decline in testosterone levels. Depression and anxiety may contribute to ED or a lack of libido, but antidepressants (such as SSRIs) may make the problem worse.

The presence of cancer and the use of chemotherapy are additional considerations. One of the symptoms of prostate cancer, which is one of the most common malignancies in males, is unexpected erectile dysfunction. Another twist on the knife is that erectile dysfunction (ED) is frequent after treatment for prostate cancer. A decrease in testosterone production is a side effect of radiation therapy for the prostate that can also impact nearby tissues, particularly the testes. Erectile dysfunction can be a side effect of surgery for pelvic malignancies, including colon cancer. Nerve injury is a potential complication of surgery. Damage to any of the nerves that supply the penis can have a devastating effect on a man's ability to maintain an erection.

HORMONES

Erections rely on a steady supply of testosterone and other hormones in the body. There are numerous factors that can disturb hormonal equilibrium. Low testosterone levels, brought on by obesity and aging, are linked to decreased libido and even erectile dysfunction. An estrogen surge might also cause problems. Although estrogen is typically associated with females, a healthy hormonal panel will also include a small amount of estrogen for men. An increase in estrogen secretion in men has been linked to both advanced age and a large percentage of abdominal obesity. This explains why guys of a certain age or weight might appear plumper or even acquire breasts. The sexual health of men can be negatively impacted by the misuse of anabolic steroids. A ripped physique is often seen as a panacea for single guys who want to impress potential spouses. The body's natural ability to produce testosterone will be damaged over time by steroid use. We have a feedback system for our hormones, so if we give ourselves some, our brains will recognize it and stop us from making any more of that hormone. Because of this, male steroid users are more likely to experience side effects such as enlarged breasts, thinning hair, smaller testicles, delayed puberty, infertility, and erectile dysfunction. As a result of today's norms in the United States, men are at a considerable disadvantage. Less physical activity on the part of men is a major contributor to their increasingly high rates of obesity. Hormonal balance is disrupted by the prevalence of processed foods in our diets, hormone-treated meat, and accidental ingestion of microplastics. The erection is the first sign of a lifetime of bad habits breaking down the body.

Lack of sleep is one factor that few guys give any thought to. While pulling an occasional all-nighter isn't a big deal, chronic sleep deprivation can have serious health consequences. Sleep plays an important role in development and repair. Testosterone is one substance that is created while you sleep. No need to be a night owl or work a lot of hours. Sleep apnea is another possible trigger for erectile dysfunction. Even if those with sleep apnea don't realize it, they're continually having their sleep interrupted. The benefits of getting 7–9 hours of sleep every night are well-documented, but in the sake of hustling, people often disregard or even despise sleep.

LIFESTYLE

ED can be exacerbated by a number of common ways of living. Smoking's negative effects on your libido should be reason enough to abandon the habit.

Nicotine inhibits nitric oxide production and disrupts the chemical cascade that NO relies on to relax smooth muscles and dilate blood vessels. As long as you refrain from lighting up again, this condition will eventually go away. While the repercussions of smoking cigarettes are generally accepted, the same cannot be said about marijuana. The scientific evidence is weak and contradictory.

The use of alcoholic beverages can potentially cause ED. Premature ejaculation, libido loss, and other sexual problems have all been linked to heavy alcohol consumption. The most well-known negative effect of alcohol, however, is the classic whisky dick, or the temporary inability to develop an erection after drinking. Some men find that drinking a little liquid courage helps them overcome their inhibitions and engage in sexual activity, but there is such a thing as too much of a good thing. Though alcohol's CNS-depressant effects can help you unwind, it comes at the expense of alert mental processing. Because of this, your brain's signal is unable to reach your penis, where it is desperately needed. Perhaps you're staring at a stunning woman and finding yourself thinking all the sexy ideas you can think in an effort to force your penis into an erection. But if that signal doesn't penetrate below the waist, it's useless.

It's possible that ED can be brought on by any of the many habits that lead to obesity. Obesity is largely caused by one's diet and lack of physical activity. Losing your self-esteem is a side effect of experiencing a physical transformation that is stigmatized by mainstream culture. Getting undressed in front of another person might be nerve-wracking if you aren't feeling up to it, and that's before you include in the weak pump, clogged and weakened pipes, and lack in endurance. This can open up a whole new can of worms that will persist despite your best efforts to treat your soft penis.

PSYCHOLOGICAL

ACCESS TO PORNOGRAPHY

The availability of porn has had a devastating effect on male wellbeing. This is not a moral condemnation of its use, but there are serious repercussions that must be discussed. As a result of seeing porn, people often develop unrealistic ideals of how men and women should seem, talk, and act. The cast guys are usually fit, well-endowed, and able (or edited) to endure more than half an hour of a co-star gushing over him, talking nasty, and being very young and very hot. There are currently billions of these videos available online. For relief from their anger and, much worse, their boredom, many men look to porn as a source of entertainment. It's understandable that spectators might experience some degree of self-doubt when presented with the opportunity to engage in sexual activity with a real live human being. Porn is acceptable, but if you need it to be aroused, you may have a problem.

DEBUNKING ERECTILE DYSFUNCTION MYTHS

When looking into ED, you could find a lot of misinformation. People looking for a quick fix are sometimes duped by "gurus" selling books and courses or by those who insist their own experience is scientific proof that the falsehoods they've heard are true. Because of catchy headlines, clickbait thumbnails, and colorful people more interested in making a quick cash than helping their fellow man, proper research, which is backed up albeit boring, is buried. Either that, or it's a way for average guys to deny that ED is a real thing that might happen to them someday. Assumptions like "that guy only acquired ED because he was old" or "he is impotent because he masturbates often" convert ED into an inevitability or, worse, a character failure, making it simple to bury one's head in the sand and ignore the problem. Particularly problematic is the use of moral reasoning to see incapacity as a matter of willpower that can be overcome by discipline rather than by seeking professional aid.

ERECTILE DYSFUNCTION IS CAUSED BY MASTURBATION

If you have erectile dysfunction and are looking for help online, you will likely read that you should stop masturbating. Essentially, this is true to some extent. Some men employ a "death grip" or far more force than they would ever use on a woman when they masturbate. The ability to expand and contract the vaginal muscles is a result of giving birth. When a woman is sexually excited, her vaginal walls dilate, making intercourse more enjoyable, and she gets moist to finish the act. We can't even come close to recreating a human vagina with our hands. It's less cozy, causes more friction (even with lotion), and can be uncomfortable if it's too tight. These combinations could dull a man's sense of pleasure from sex and lead to erectile dysfunction. It is recommended that you learn more effective methods of masturbation, but not that you stop doing it altogether. It goes against human nature, and there are no studies to back it up. Masturbation is an essential human trait.

Animals as diverse as dogs and monkeys engage in masturbation. It's not a sign of weakness or lack of self-control; it's a normal part of being human. It's good for men's sexual health and a great way to release extra energy if it's done in moderation.

Men are drawn to the no-fap movement on the internet because they believe it will help them with their erectile dysfunction. Videos will show them how giving up sexual pleasure improved their lives, got rid of their ED, and made them more useful citizens. In truth, it's dangerously close to being a cult. Forum where men boast about spending months or years without masturbating. The majority of these groups' leaders feed off of the insecurity brought on by ED. They try to sell books or courses, and if a student fails to meet expectations, they are made to feel bad about themselves. Humans are perfectly capable of healthy masturbation. Forget about giving it up altogether; doing so won't help you beat ED.

PHYSICAL DEPENDENCE ON VIAGRA IS INEVITABLE

The worry that they'll need the drug every time they want to have sex for the rest of their lives is another factor that makes guys reluctant to use medication. Having sex before going to the pharmacy can be intimidating and demeaning to men. Maintaining an erection may no longer be a problem if you've resolved the underlying physical or psychological factor that was making it difficult for you to do so without Viagra. It appears that this concern is limited to issues of mental and sexual well-being solely. It's inappropriate to question someone with diabetes whether they're worried about becoming insulin-dependent. Medication use, whether short- or long-term, should be treated with no shame. You're already struggling, so taking this medicine won't make things any worse. By following a straightforward prescription, you can lead a regular, secure sex life.

ERECTILE DYSFUNCTION IS SOMETHING ONLY OLD PEOPLE GET

There is a common misconception about the kinds of guys that experience ED. Most of the time, it's the elderly who are shown dragging themselves to the doctor while the rest of us chuckle at their dilemma in the media. True, the prevalence of ED is rising, and it's now being diagnosed in younger men. The accumulation of age-related diseases, like heart disease and diabetes, is the strongest predictor of erectile dysfunction, not age itself. Access to pornography, gorgeous women on their social media feeds, and beliefs about masculinity can increase anxiety around sex, though this is less common in younger guys. In other words, if you maintain your healthy lifestyle as you age, you won't be doomed to ED. A man's lifestyle choices may have unanticipated repercussions. Poor food, inactivity, sleep deprivation, and mental illness can have negative impacts on males at any age.

Men tend to be very critical of themselves when it comes to sex difficulties. In this situation, neither person has any clothing on and neither person is in complete command of what happens. Women have their own sex troubles, but it is not as socially stigmatized if they are too tight or can't orgasm as it is if a guy has the same problem. Orgasming is a time-consuming process for women, therefore normal PIV sex requires an erection. The fear of being exposed and defenseless is exacerbated by the fact that, without an erection, the party is over. As fewer people engage in sexual activity on a regular basis, it's changed from being something to look forward to to being something to worry about.

INFERTILITY AND ERECTILE DYSFUNCTION ARE SYNONYMOUS.

Some people mistakenly believe that if a man has ED, he is also sterile. Although ED makes it more challenging to actually get a woman pregnant, it has no bearing on the quality of the sperm. One can have both normal sperm production and erectile dysfunction in a male. Low sperm counts are the primary cause of infertility. Infertility can interfere with a man's ability to get hard, and this worry is real. Once more, sexual activity is viewed in a bad light. A man's inability to father a child and the challenges he faces in establishing his marriage can leave him feeling diminished. As relationship issues go, the desire to start a family and the prospect of having children of one's own rank near the top. To have one's own children, one must not be willing to make many concessions. It's the one thing every human being wants, and if he can't have them, it can screw with his sense of self-worth.

ERECTILE DYSFUNCTION IS AN AZZ OR NOTHING PHENOMENON

Even if you've been diagnosed with erectile dysfunction, you could still be able to get an erection occasionally. You should see a urologist if it interferes with your sexual life. If a man can get an erection on occasion or has no trouble finishing a masturbation session on his own, he may not suspect he has erectile dysfunction. If a man has even sporadic success in keeping an erection going, he is even less likely to seek treatment. They can just deny that anything serious is going on, and the whole thing is embarrassing for them anyway. However, you can rest assured that any doctor worth their salt would never pass judgment on a patient for asking a reasonable question regarding their health. At the very least, they will value the heads-up that anything is off with their patient's health and well-being.

CHAPTER 2

THE HISTORY OF TREATING ERECTILE DYSFUNCTION

Male impotence has been a problem for mankind since since it first emerged. People have been trying to figure out how to have an erection since ancient times. The history of the word "impotence" demonstrates that this is and always has been an issue. Lack of authority in Latin is a reflection of how little masculine expectations have changed over time. Witchcraft, divine intervention, demons, and having sex with "undesirable women" were once considered potential causes of impotence before medical science uncovered the role of the circulatory system and the mind. The inability of a man to have sex with his wife was considered one of the few grounds for divorce. In Medieval France, males who faced charges of impotence were required to demonstrate their ability to keep an erection for the court. In those days, impotence was really punishable by law. Women weren't always the ones who benefited from it.

Several women were executed during the Salem witch trials on charges of practicing witchcraft with the intent to render a man sterile. Masturbation was held responsible for ED in Victorian times, which is understandable given the era's more puritanical social norms. Having the ability to have sexual encounters is a huge burden, so it's not surprising that many researchers have spent their careers trying to discover a way to alleviate it.

WACKY "CURES" FOR NOT GETTING IT UP

Some genuinely odd solutions arose in the search for the cure (or at least something that gullible men would believe was a cure). In order to stimulate sexual desire, ancient cultures typically rubbed a mixture of plants. Complicated concoctions were developed to either rub on the penis or ingest, and they typically included a number of different herbs, beans, and honey. Acupuncture was promoted by the Chinese as a treatment for impotence. As if teaching his students how to cook wasn't enough, a Tunisian man named Al Jazzar also gave them the incredible remedy of caressing, kissing, good words, and finding happiness with their relationship.

All the testicles of all the endangered species have been turned into a soup for the treatment of impotence at some time. Another popular treatment involved mixing bull urine with dirt. Still, the widespread use of animal components in medical treatments is a major cause for concern. Traditional medicine typically relies on the organs of more common animals like mice and goats, but it has also been known to use testicles from tigers, shark fins, seal penis, the contents of whale intestines, seahorses, toad skin glands, and antlers. Baby alligator hearts were crushed and used in ancient Egyptian medicine. All the testicles of all the endangered species have been turned into a soup for the treatment of impotence at some time.

This outlook was not exclusive to antiquated medical practices. In the West, an extract made from sheep testicles was widely used as a treatment for impotence. There were plenty of snake oil sellers promising to treat male impotence, and even more men who believed them. John Brinkley, one of the people who thought those treatments were inadequate, said so. Instead, he charged current equivalent of $10,000 to implant goat testicle glands into male patients. Brinley advertised the procedure as if it were a revolutionary breakthrough, citing the amazing Billy the goat kid whose father had the procedure. This operation was useless at best, and it led to terrible infections and permanent damage at worst. Eventually, Brindley's medical license was revoked and he died in poverty, but his legacy as a charlatan in the field of medicine lives on to this day.

With the development of pharmacology and the introduction of crude penis pumps and implants in the 20th century, the nightmare of treatment gradually faded. The solution to a man's impotence problem may lie in a change in diet, according to some claims. When advertising a diet to males, a boost in sexual vitality is a common selling point.

Furthermore, there is a common misconception that consuming phallic-shaped foods would improve erections.

Then in 1992, a major development occurred. Pfizer researchers were developing a drug to alleviate angina symptoms in patients. Many research participants experienced erections as a side effect of the medication, but the drug did not have the desired effect on chest pain. Pfizer saw a golden opportunity in this finding and shifted their focus from cardiovascular to sexual health. Which eventually led to the development of Viagra. In 1998, it was the first ED drug to clear the FDA's rigorous approval process. Since then, its effects on pharmaceuticals have grown to the point where it can be considered a phenomenon. The trademark blue color and brand name make it easy to identify. Viagra is the most popular erectile dysfunction drug despite the availability of Cialis, Stendra, and Staxyn.

CHAPTER 3

WHAT 15 VIAGRA AND HOW DOES IT WORK?

In short, Viagra is a small blue pill that widens blood vessels and improves blood flow. To achieve an erection, Viagra blocks the action of phosphodiesterase type 5, an enzyme that degrades cyclic guanosine monophosphate (cGMP) in excess. Cialis and Levitra are two other PED5 inhibitors. If you want it to be effective, you need to wait at least half an hour before engaging in sexual activity. Because the body is unable to degrade cGMP and the blood vessels are opened, the natural cascade that leads to an erection is magnified to the point where a man who previously had trouble keeping an erection may have a regular sex life.

OBTAINING A PRESCRIPTION

Viagra requires a visit to the doctor to address erectile problems before a prescription can be written. It's not OTC because it depends on things like a person's medical history and the medicines they're already taking. A lot of questions will be asked regarding your sexual health and the difficulties you're having during the session. Your sexual desire and the length of your erections, if you can get them, will be tracked. Also, during a physical examination, your penis and testicles may be inspected for any outward signs of dysfunction, such as diminished size or discolored blood vessels. You might also have your chest measured to see whether it's abnormally big, which could mean your testosterone and estrogen levels are off. Regular erections are an excellent indicator of men's health, therefore the doctor may order blood tests to rule out diabetes and other conditions. They'll take your vitals and conduct a heart evaluation as well. Your mental health may also be investigated. Although many guys prefer to keep their cool when discussing this delicate subject, being open and honest is the key to receiving effective treatment.

There may be more involved or lengthy steps involved in an ED diagnosis, depending on the circumstances. Overnight Test of Erectile Function. Keep in mind that having several erections during sleep is completely common for men. The penis is probed with this gadget, and the number of erections a guy gets while sleeping is recorded. In addition, this can assist determine whether a person's ED is a result of a psychological or physiological issue.

A physician may prescribe an Injection Test to see if there is a problem with blood flow to the penis. You should not count on getting this examination. An erection-inducing drug is injected directly into the corpus cavernosa of a healthy male. A problem with blood supply to the penis should be investigated if it doesn't. When combined with a Doppler Ultrasound Test, this method allows for an in-depth analysis of the penis's anatomical make-up and blood flow. The doctor will also check to see if the erection is painful or if the penis has become curled (Peyronie's Disease) during the injection.

You will be prescribed Viagra once your doctor has given you the all-clear to do so. You will most likely be prescribed a daily pill of 50 milligrams (mg). With a half-life of only 3–4 hours, this medication is best taken once daily and never shared with another person. If it doesn't work, talk to your doctor about increasing your dosage of Viagra to 100 mg. While Viagra is widely known, it is important to take many precautions before and while using the pill.

CONTRAINDICATIONS

Doctors are reluctant to prescribe Viagra for a variety of reasons. There are situations where the potential side effects of the medicine might be too great to justify. The medicine can't be taken if you aren't physically able to have sex. Viagra won't make every man strong and masculine, unfortunately. Viagra is recommended for men of senior age, however a man's decreasing health may prevent him from using the drug. Age-related kidney and liver problems are not always incompatible with treatment, but they can modify both the recommended dosage and the patient's ability to tolerate the drug. Although the list of Viagra's contraindications is broad and constantly evolving, the following have long been included:

- Advanced kidney disease
- Advance liver disease
- Angina

- **Certain arrhythmias**
- Certain eye conditions
- Chronic low blood pressure
- Congestive heart failure
- Heart attack
- Leukemia
- Multiple myeloma

- Peyronie's disease (or having a bent penis when erect)
- Sickle Cell disease
- Stroke
- Uncontrolled high blood pressure

THE VIAGRA ALTERNATIVE

Viagra and similar medications are prescribed to men who may or may not have erectile dysfunction. Pulmonary hypertension is an example of such a condition. Pulmonary hypertension is characterized by an elevation of blood pressure within the pulmonary arteries. As a result, you may have trouble breathing, have swelling in your limbs, feel lightheaded, or even pass out. Sildenafil has been utilized as an adjunctive therapy in the treatment of this illness, albeit it is not the sole option. As a vasodilator, it can be useful for treating pulmonary hypertension and its associated symptoms. While it is the same medication, it will not be sold under the Viagra brand name. To be branded as Revatio.

Raynaud Syndrome is yet another medical ailment that can benefit from Viagra-like treatments. Caused by a total closure of the arterioles, blood supply is cut off to the extremities. Although the illness causes a total whiteout of the fingers, it is otherwise quite benign (though there is a risk of gangrene). Given that this is a cardiovascular problem, sildenafil can be prescribed off-label to widen the arterioles and improve blood flow.

An interesting aside is that Viagra works wonders on floral arrangements. Flowers benefit from reduced cGMP breakdown since it allows them to flourish for longer.

WHAT VIAGRA IS NOT

Fear of starting Viagra had Jim feeling anxious. After some basic health checks and an examination, he was given the necessary medication. He wanted to be optimistic, but doubts kept popping up. He blamed advancing age for his erectile dysfunction, but admitted that marital issues had contributed to the issue. Since he and his wife constantly argued and started viewing one other less as partners, the bedroom became sterile. Still, he hoped that if they revived their sexual relationship, everything else would return to normal. Jim was prepared to give everything a shot for the sake of his family, even if he and his partner just couldn't seem to get on the same page. Jim was disappointed to find that after taking the tablet and waiting for half an hour, nothing had happened. The next day, he called his doctor, but the physician did not have an answer to his predicament. After years of marital discord, Jim realized he was no longer physically attracted to his wife after doing some research on online forums about dead bedrooms. A jolt of truth hit me like ice water. Viagra and pornography helped Jim get an erection, but his real-life wife still failed to do the trick.

The inability to maintain an erection is a frustrating condition for most guys. They are looking for a quick fix so they may go on with their lives. Even if the medicine does what it's supposed to, many people will have unrealistic expectations because of this. The inability of the penis to fill with and retain blood is an issue that Viagra helps men with. This is not an aphrodisiac. It's only a mechanical fix that won't make your lover any more beautiful or boost your libido. Arousal is a prerequisite for its effectiveness. A drug will not be effective if there is a mental barrier to its full effect. If this is happening, you should talk to a doctor rather than giving up or increasing your dose in the vain belief that the problem lies with the dosage.

Due to the complex nature of the factors that contribute to erectile dysfunction, Viagra is not a magic bullet for many people. In order to permanently beat ED, you must also deal with its root cause. Viagra is a helpful tool for overcoming some physical obstacles. The effectiveness of Viagra could decrease over time if the underlying problems deteriorate.

YOUR MARRIAGE MAY NOT BE SAVED BY THIS.

Pride, vulnerability, sexual expectations, gendered expectations, and communication are all potential stumbling blocks in a sexually dysfunctional relationship. No amount of Viagra will save your marriage if the issue isn't mechanical; conversely, even if it is, saving it will require open lines of communication and mutual understanding. While many couples use Viagra successfully, some spouses may find the concept offensive. The very act of introducing it might make people feel insecure and even angry. Having to rely on medication to fix the plumbing can make one partner feel insufficient. Because having sex now feels like an appointment or planned event, this could be seen as a barrier. Since it takes Viagra 30 minutes to 1 hour to take effect, you'll have to sacrifice the thrill of unplanned sex as a result. When you put it that way, the allure of sex is diminished.

When men take Viagra, there is a risk that they will begin to think and act in abnormal ways towards sexuality and romantic partnerships. They may feel ashamed of their reliance on the little blue pill for even the most fundamental social interactions, and this insecurity may appear in various ways within their relationships. Since the pill can be costly, another concern is that some men feel pressured to "get their money's worth" each time they take it. You can't pay for a sex experience that doesn't feel worth your time and effort, so make sure it's spectacular, lasts a while, and includes some risk-taking. It's stressful for the couple because they can't control each other's timetables. A partner may feel guilty if they suddenly want to back out before the Viagra kicks in. That's a really risky sex dynamic, yet it's real for some Viagra users.

Many assumptions are made about the pill, including that it will increase a man's libido, his enjoyment, and his luck with the ladies. Given how Viagra is marketed, this viewpoint is to be expected. In ads, men and women are shown to be "content" while a catchy tune (Viva Viagra!) plays in the background. The ads feature middle-aged men who appear to be quite successful, all of whom are smiling and enjoying the company of much younger and more attractive women. These promises are effective at getting people to part with their cash, but they may do incredible harm.

CHAPTER 4
THINGS YOU SHOULD KNOW BEFORE TAKING VIAGRA

Taking Viagra safely is essential if it is to be an effective treatment for your erectile dysfunction. Despite the seemingly humorous and carefree side effects of Viagra, the drug should not be treated lightly. It's possible to experience negative effects, abuse it, or eventually have to stop taking it for health reasons.

COMMON SIDE EFFECTS OF VIAGRA

Most people who take Viagra experience only minor, temporary negative effects. Among them are

- Changes in vision
- Dizziness
- Flushing or redness
- Headache
- Light sensitivity
- Nausea
- Upset stomach

These reactions are common, as blood pressure lowers significantly when using Viagra. Imagine a large container full of water. There will be a lot of pressure because you have one tank full to capacity. Once you transfer the same volume of water to a different container, the pressure will decrease. When our blood arteries dilate, our container simply expands to accommodate more fluid. It's important to keep tabs on these symptoms, but they likely won't need medical attention. However, if they get worse while using Viagra, you should talk to your doctor right away.

NEGATIVE REPERCUSSIONS THAT CAN OCCUR VERY INFREQUENTLY

Commercials for Viagra can be humorous up to the point where the drug's long list of potential adverse effects is read. Of course, it's important to point out that the infrequent but severe adverse effects are worth discussing. Although most guys are content with their meds, it's still important to provide them all the info they need to make an informed choice.

VISION LOSS

Viagra has been linked to blindness and visual loss in a small number of male users. Low blood pressure neuropathy can alter or distort one's vision. Some guys who take Viagra end up with a detachment of their retinas. The idea of having sex so good that it blinds you is appealing, but if you take Viagra and find that your eyesight has blurred, you should stop taking it and consult a doctor. This is probably only a momentary thing, but you should see a doctor anyhow.

LOSS OF HEARING

While the exact mechanism is unknown, Viagra has been linked to cases of permanent hearing loss. Dizziness and ringing in the ears are possible side effects. At this time, it is thought that the pill's increased blood flow can travel to the ears, where it could potentially harm the auditory system's sensitive network. More study is necessary, however this is a rare but real possibility when taking ED drugs.

"IF YOUR ERECTIONS LASTS FOR MORE THAN FOUR HOURS, SEEK MEDICAL ATTENTION IMMEDIATELY"

Each and every time this sentence appears at the end of a Viagra commercial, it elicits a range of responses from the audience. Some people might think this is fantastic, after all, who wouldn't enjoy a sex-filled marathon? This, however, is a legitimate worry that can result in long-term consequences. This condition is known in the medical community as priapism. Nothing is entertaining about a medical situation in which the penis remains erect for hours on end. For men who suffer with it, the pain can be unbearable. The penis becomes physically incapable of releasing the blood, therefore no amount of pressure will ever bring it down from its full mast position. Men may avoid medical attention for this issue for several hours or even days because of its potential for embarrassment. This may cause irreversible damage, making it impossible for the male to get an erection again. In the extremely unlikely event that you experience this issue, you should seek immediate medical attention. It's unlikely that the doctors there will react negatively to or make fun of priapism, as they have seen it all before.

CONTRAINDICATIONS AND INTERACTIONS BETWEEN DRUGS

Before beginning Viagra, your medications should be carefully reviewed. You should consult your doctor before beginning Viagra treatment if you are already taking medicine for the treatment of a condition that affects your ability to maintain an erection (something you know a lot about after reading this book). Relevant drug categories include:

Hypertension medication e Nitrates

PDE5 inhibitors

Prescription nitrates intended to improve cardiovascular health are the most common cause of adverse effects. If you're experiencing chest pain, your doctor may recommend nitroglycerin. Because it dilates blood arteries, it also provides relief from the symptoms of heart disease. Fainting, a hazardous drop in blood pressure, and headaches are possible side effects of taking two of these pills at once. If you have high blood pressure, you may find that some drugs, such as alpha-blockers and those for pulmonary hypertension, interact with Viagra and increase its effects.

There is also the potential for trouble with antifungals and antibiotics including Lefamulin, Erythromycin, and Voxelotor. However, it can slow Viagra's breakdown in the body, which can lead to some toxicity, albeit it does not interact with Viagra in the same manner as hypertension does.

When combined with some HIV antivirals like Norvir, Viagra can cause a number of undesirable side effects. It has the potential to interact with Viagra and increase its effects to dangerous levels. You must be open and honest with your doctor about your medical and drug history, even though this is a lengthy and annoying list. It is fine to wait to obtain cleared for Viagra if you are only using these drugs momentarily. If you don't, though, there are many other options for dealing with ED that should meet your needs.

OTHER INTERACTIONS

ALCOHOL

A dangerous interaction between alcohol and Viagra is possible. Consuming alcohol in moderation is safe, but it may lessen the efficacy of medications like Viagra. Whisky dick is a well-known side effect of alcohol because to the depressant effects of alcohol on the neurological system and the dehydrating effects of whisky. So, even if Viagra does its job, there may not be enough fluid in the body to keep an erection going. It increases the risk of unpleasant side effects without adding any benefit. Therefore, it is not recommended to combine Viagra with alcoholic beverages.

GRAPEFRUIT

There are a number of drugs that don't get along well with grapefruit or grapefruit juice. Grapefruit inhibits the intestinal metabolism of drugs. It's counterintuitive, but because the body isn't breaking down the medication, the blood concentration of the drug actually increases. This is because the entire dose is absorbed into the bloodstream more rapidly. At first glance, this may sound promising, as it suggests that grapefruit may enhance the efficacy and duration of Viagra. Because your doctor has given you a specific dosage for a reason, doing so is extremely risky. There is a higher chance of undesirable side effects as well. Grapefruit juice should be avoided whole, not only before taking Viagra.

CHAPTER 5

OTHER FACTORS THAT CAN IMPROVE ERECTILE DYSFUNCTION

Healthy sexual health encompasses much more than just the mechanics of an erection. The only way to effectively treat erectile dysfunction is to address not just the symptoms, but also any underlying causes. You will not only improve your sex life but also extend it.

EXERCISE

Even if you aren't aware of the benefits, starting an exercise routine will greatly improve your sexual life. The benefits of aerobic exercise on heart health are numerous. You'll have healthy blood flow and clear arteries thanks to this. The mechanical cause of ED can be mitigated with a regular exercise routine, and the benefits extend far beyond that. Regular exercise will improve your stamina for all the physical activity required in sex. In addition, it causes the production of dopamine and other "feel-good" hormones, making it an effective treatment for mental illness. Improving one's physical health also boosts confidence. Hitting the gym, the track, or the trails will help you feel and look great.

DIET

When you consider how much exercise helps with ED, it's not surprising that eating well can help the sections below as well. Those with diabetes can benefit the most from a weight loss plan that also promotes a healthy weight. When undesirable fat is lost, the body's hormonal and metabolic profiles can improve, and the cardiovascular system benefits. Most well-rounded diets support these aims, although research into specific components and diets has shown promise in reducing the symptoms of ED. One such diet is the Mediterranean diet. Fruits, vegetables, olive oil, legumes, and whole grains all play prominent roles in this diet. Red meat, processed foods, alcohol, and refined carbohydrates are also off-limits on the regimen. Additionally investigated foods include: Celery Garlic Ginger Ginseng Root of Maca Vitamin D supplements

This further illustrates what has been stressed many times over. You can't have a good erection if your physique isn't in good shape. Medication is helpful, but the advantages of a healthy lifestyle cannot be overstated.

THERAPY

All guys should take care of their emotional health just as much as their physical health. Many guys put off attending to their mental health in the hopes that they may find a magic bullet that would prevent them from having to face their problems head-on. When a psychogenic factor, such anxiety, contributes to ED, it's in the patient's best interest to address the source of their distress. The help of a skilled sex therapist, cognitive behavioral therapy, or the adoption of coping mechanisms like meditation can restore a man's sense of stability. The goal of sexual activity is to have fun and show affection for one another. Many guys have completely lost it, whether out of fear of hurting their partner's feelings, embarrassment, or unfair expectations. Confiding in an objective bystander can help you organize your chaotic sexual ideas into something more manageable for analysis. Putting your anxieties into words is a vital step toward facing and overcoming them.

TO LIVEN UP YOUR SEXUAL EXPERIENCE

Trying something new in the bedroom can be stimulating for both partners. Most people only think about the climax, however sex has many other wonderful aspects. The trip itself is more important than any final objective. When you know you have options than penile erection, penetration becomes less intimidating. Even without a penis, a woman can experience an orgasmic climax using her fingers, toys, and tongue. Any effort to "beat" impotence into submission will end in frustration for both partners. Adding new features and postures will help you rediscover your erogenous side if you've noticed your sex life becoming more formulaic. Anything that can turn sex into a positive experience rather than a negative one is welcome.

Also problematic are acts like masturbation and pornographic media. Cutting back if you find yourself dependent on it could be helpful, especially if you don't have a partner to engage in sex with, but refraining entirely is not the solution. To get your penis used to responding to a lighter grasp, you'll need to be more mindful of your technique. Neither of you are competing in a race. Be patient, entertain sexy thoughts, and savor the anticipation. Keep it relaxed if you find yourself clenching your fists or using excessive force in your strokes. The typical individual doesn't get a very accurate depiction of sex from the mainstream porn that's aimed at males. It's usually rather hostile and humiliating to everyone involved. It's a mass-produced item used to induce fast erections in men. Many buyers of the product are embarrassed by the content of the films they watch, but the industry keeps cranking up the intensity until the content is unrecognizable as sex. A partner's animosity will grow if vanilla suddenly stops working. Having kinks is not something to be ashamed of, but it might reduce your options and leave sex feeling unfulfilling and unpleasant. Look for erotica in a variety of places, including those that specifically cater to women. Although it's not at all like what you're used to, it may help you see sexuality in a new light. Being able to appreciate what women value from their perspective can make sexual encounters much more enjoyable.

OPTIONS TO VIAGRA

For many men, Viagra is not the answer. Men may not be able to participate due to physical or mental health concerns, and that's fine. The fact that this is the most commonly cited answer does not imply that it is the only viable option. If you have an intolerance to Viagra but are able to take other PDE5 inhibitors, you have options outside Viagra. It's possible to take some of them by just dissolving them under the tongue.

There are alternatives to taking pills. Men who have no tolerance for medication may benefit from using vacuum equipment. With the help of a pump, blood is pumped to the penis and held in place by a ring. The erection it delivers is gratifying, and there are almost no negative consequences. When contemporary drugs are ineffective, it can be an excellent cure if used by someone who has been trained in its use and is ready to forego spontaneity. In addition to the aforementioned medications, there are also common wearable devices that can help you keep (rather than get) an erection. Their effectiveness relies on creating tension, which, while it might extend the pleasure of sex, can be unpleasant for those who aren't accustomed to it. Real implants that are inserted into the penis are another option. A scrotal pump that can be controlled manually to produce an erection is involved. If something seems extreme, that's because it is. Due to the intrusive nature of surgery and the inherent hazards involved, it is only done as a last resort when other treatments have failed.

Injections are an additional viable option. Injectable medications like Caverject work by stimulating blood flow to the penile erector muscle. Most guys, unfortunately, will be unwilling to risk injecting anything into such a sensitive place. However, if used correctly and the fear of needles is conquered, it may be a tremendous aid in your sex life.

Many men, especially older ones, fail to consider testosterone replacement therapy as a viable alternative. And if your doctor approves, it can do wonders for your sex life as well as your physical health and looks. When used to counteract the gradual decline in testosterone that occurs with age, it can effectively reverse the effects of time. Despite its increasing popularity, more research into the potential dangers of this trend is warranted. Inasmuch as it targets hormones, there is always a chance of cancer recurrence. As you can see, having ED does not have to be a permanent condition.

CONCLUSION

Erectile Dysfunction is a multidimensional issue that can be stressful for many people globally. Men no longer have to wear the testicles of an endangered animal as a talisman or put their faith in medical quacks peddling snake oil or talismans thanks to Viagra and other ED treatments. Since the introduction of Viagra, men's sex lives and self-esteems have improved. Men of any age and dealing with a wide range of problems can benefit from this method of regaining their mojo.

However, it's crucial to retain a level head and realistic expectations about how far Viagra can go in overcoming sexual inhibitions. Not only will it not make you more attractive or improve your libido, but it also won't spare you from the hell that is divorce court. It's a great answer to one problem, but you'll have to figure out the rest on your own. Effective communication, finding mental health resources, and being realistic about sex and the pill will go a long way in enhancing your relationships and your self-esteem. If the capacity to get and keep an erection helps you become a more daring and assured lover, then you are becoming the finest version of yourself, not the pill. The erection may have been a contributing factor, but if you still feel uneasy, unattracted to your spouse, that sex is a chore, or that it causes you anxiety, then you need to address underlying issues if you want a good sex life. It is crucial to parse out these concerns before giving up hope totally.

Maintaining a healthy state of mind and body is essential for a fulfilling sexual life, especially as you become older. Since ED is caused by underlying health problems, avoiding such problems in the first place can eliminate the need for Viagra altogether. Maintaining an erection into old age is facilitated by exercise, avoiding a sedentary lifestyle, and eating well. Viagra is a viable tool for individuals who are healthy enough for it, but nothing will replace a regimen that will maintain all areas of your body healthy. Keep in mind that a healthy heart is required to transport all that blood below.

Keeping your erection is a fantastic motivation and a great reward for maintaining overall wellness. If Viagra helps you feel more confident and positive, which in turn motivates you to take care of your health as a whole, then there's no reason to feel guilty about using it. A man's capacity to look at an issue objectively and employ all available means to solve it, including the use of medication, is a commendable trait, not a sign of weakness. No amount of willpower is going to work here; you'll need medical intervention or medication. There is no shame in trying Viagra if you believe it would help. To be the healthiest and greatest version of yourself, discuss your options with your doctor.

NOTE

END

CPSIA information can be obtained
at www.ICGtesting.com
Printed in the USA
LVHW081555080123
736722LV00029B/450